Natural Methods to Prevent and Treat Alzheimer's

By: Alyson Rodgers

Published by:
Alyson Rodgers and Random Technologies
4409 HOFFNER AVENUE, SUITE 347
Belle Isle, FL 32812

Disclaimer

This guide has been written to offer educational information to individuals suffering from Alzheimer's, or at risk of Alzheimer's. To that end, it is meant to be used as a *guide*, not a substitute for professional medical advice or doctor visits.

If you are currently being treated for Alzheimer's or ADRD, do not discontinue that treatment without first seeking the advice of the medical professional who initiated treatment.

By reading this guide, you agree to the fact that the author and publisher cannot and will not be held responsible for any side effects that occur through the use or misuse of the advice provided in this book.

I will be providing a lot of information to help, but I do want to be clear that all of my research still does not amount to a medical degree – and it should not be treated like it does. That being said, enjoy the book, and feel free to implement the treatments – after seeking approval from a medically qualified healthcare professional.

Table of Contents

Natural Methods for Prevention and Treatment of Alzheimer's 1

Where Did We Find Alzheimer's Anyway?.....................................3

What is Alzheimer's 5

What Makes Alzheimer's Different From Dementia?.....................7

Identifying Alzheimer's...8

The Progression of Alzheimer's – Stages to Watch For 10

Potential Causes of Alzheimer's..16

Does Genetics Play A Role In Alzheimer's? 18

Treating Alzheimer's 20

    Experimental Drugs? 23

    NonSteroidal Anti-Inflammatory Drugs (NSAIDs).................25

Prevention, Not Treatment 27

There Are Natural Methods Too! 29

    Antioxidants...32

    Alpha Lipoic Acid (ALA)...33

    Acetyl-L-Carnitine (ALC)..34

    Boron – And How to Use It Safely..35

    Curry..36

    Ginkgo Biloba..37

    Huperzia Serrata (Huperzine)..38

    Lecithin..39

    Vitamins C & E...40

    Zinc..42

General Health of Your Brain and Body 43

    Omega 3 Fatty Acids 44

    Vitamin B Family 45

Why Worry About The Brain Anyway?..46

What You DON'T Want In Your body 48

    Aluminum...49

    Mercury 50

    Alcohol and Nicotine – The Bad Guys in Most Health Food
    Guides...51

    High Cholesterol...53

    Research Controversy about High Cholesterol....................56

    Controlling Your Cholesterol Levels – Should you be On a Statin
    drug? 57

Does Meat Contribute To Alzheimer's? 58

The Importance of Eating Organic...60

The Importance of Education...62

How to Work Out Your Brain...64

The Importance of Exercise 66

Stress Reduction...69

Summary of Alzheimer's Prevention Tips.....................................71

Making a Plan to Prevent Alzheimer's..75

If You Already Have Alzheimer's, or Think You Do......................76

A 30 Day Plan to Preventing Alzheimer's.....................................78

Natural Methods for Prevention and Treatment of Alzheimer's

North American society has spent a lot of time, energy, and money on developing research around what happens to us as we age. The findings can look discouraging, with the risks ever increasing for stroke, heart disease, and other 'normal signs of aging'. But these are not the only things research has found!

Consider what the last century has done for longevity, we are living two (and sometimes three) times as long as we used to be expected to – well into our 80s and beyond! This is great, but it does bring up the opportunity for dementia to strike (in all its nasty ways).

The great news is that there are things you can do to combat the onset of dementia, or indeed Alzheimer's. By working to eat right, staying active, and generally seeking to become (and remain) healthy, you will be well on your way to the healthy happy golden years we all desire.

It's important to recognize the place of mental health in healthy aging. You are more than just your body. The mind needs just as much help to maintain itself as the body does, but is all too often neglected. This guide is going to teach you a bit about how the brain comes into play with the prevention and treatment of Alzheimer's, and walk you through understanding what's happening in your body. This guide is going to walk you through tips to a healthier lifestyle, physically and mentally.

I'll focus on teaching you more than just the physical side of Alzheimer's, because there is much more to understand about it. Alzheimer's does affect the body, but it also affects the mind, and even affects our social life and general sense of well being. Our friendships and our family will suffer alongside us, which is why it's so important to work to do everything you can to keep yourself healthy – to keep their suffering to a minimum too, but also to enable you to maintain your social life as well as your physical and mental skills.

Anything worth doing is worth doing right, and I'm going to propose that doing something right begins with making a plan. The plan this guide is meant to begin is the plan to make you healthier, by teaching you the basics of how to care for both your mind and body.

I provide you with a 30 day plan here, but this is meant to be a lifestyle changing guide.

Finally, I want to reassure you. Anyone can read this book and benefit from it. Whether you're 22 or 67, you should be working to maintain your mental health!

Where Did We Find Alzheimer's Anyway?

Alzheimer's was first recognized as a disease in 1907, due to the work of Dr. Alois Alzheimer (go figure). He was performing an autopsy on a patient and found tangled neurons within her brain, one of the indicators of Alzheimer's. Curious as a true scientist often is, Dr. Alzheimer investigated the tangles and resulting Alzheimer's plaque, and published his findings under the topic of "pre-senile dementia" in a recognized medical journal of his day.

In this time period, aging was naturally assumed to be a journey headed towards senility, the loss of ones mind and ability to remember things or take care of oneself. He thus referred to the woman as "pre-senile dementia" because although she was gradually deteriorating, she was only 51 years old – making the onset irregular and the cause for recognition.

In today's society, we are able to recognize this onset as Alzheimer's Disease (AD), and understand that not every one experiences it – although incidences of Alzheimer's are on the rise. Contemporary research has shown that there are at least 4.5 million people currently suffering from Alzheimer's in America, up from 2.25 million in just 1960.

The good news is that, thanks to Dr. Alzheimer's work and the work of many other hardworking individuals who have come since, we are able to recognize Alzheimer's, and have started working towards preventing it from happening.

This book is going to review the evidence and let you know the tried and true ways to work to help those you love.

Alzheimer's doesn't yet have a cure, but we can work to treat it – even before we fully understand what's caused it.

What is Alzheimer's

Alzheimer's disease is a condition that primarily affects ones cognitive abilities, specifically seeming to target memory. This plays out in a lack of ability to take care of oneself (forgetting you turned the stove on risking fire, forgetting where you are and winding up lost) without supervision and extra help.

Unfortunately, so far there is no cure for Alzheimer's, though there are ways to treat the symptoms and enable its victims to lead a more normal life than previously thought. Treating the symptoms of AD can increase the lifespan of the sufferer, ease the burden of caring for a loved one on friends and family, and increase the quality of life for the diagnosed individual.

Interestingly, there is no concrete method of diagnosing Alzheimer's until after death, at autopsy. This is because the signs of Alzheimer's are primarily locked away deep within the brain, in the form of these neural tangles and plaque build ups. This does not stop us from trying however.

When Alzheimer's is suspected, medical professionals begin administering scientific tests – to identify the presence of symptoms we primarily associate with Alzheimer's. Diagnosis and then treatment usually kicks in when we see symptoms themselves, but the truth is it is far better to start preparing for AD sooner than when the symptoms are visible.

How can we do that? Neural imaging.

Alzheimer's begins to tip its hand in the years leading up to its exhibition of symptoms. For some people, symptoms appear as early as age 40, and others it will not appear until they're well into their 80s. The point is to identify these symptoms within the mind as soon as possible, so you can start treating earlier than later – as is always an easier thing to do.

What Makes Alzheimer's Different From Dementia?

A lot of people can get confused from time to time between Alzheimer's and dementia. Both are conditions that impair the memory, and both are conditions that result in a loss of independence – requiring full time care after onset.

Diseases that share symptoms with Alzheimer's
- Depression
- Hypothyroidism
- Lou Gehrig's disease
- Malnutrition
- Parkinson's disease
- Stroke
- Subdural hematoma (bleeding in the brain)
- Substance abuse
- Tumors

Misdiagnosis can happen, but by carefully keeping track of the patient's symptoms and following up with a medical professional, you decrease your risk. Medical professionals are well aware of the overlap between these diseases and health issues, and they know what makes them differ – and thus how to tell the difference.

Thus, the best way to ensure that you or your loved one gets properly cared for is to track the symptoms, and seek professional medical advice if you're suspecting Alzheimer's is what's causing the changes.

Identifying Alzheimer's

Alzheimer's requires testing to be definitively diagnosed, and indeed cannot be 100% diagnosed until after death, but the medical profession is largely capable of predicting when an individual has Alzheimer's.

For this prediction to occur however, the individual has to seek out testing. This can be a problem with Alzheimer's patients, as they tend to be suffering from a) memory loss (making it harder to schedule and keep appointments) and b) shame surrounding the onset of their symptoms.

There is no reason to be ashamed if you think that you, or someone you love, is suffering from Alzheimer's! You are not alone! The key is to talk to that person in a loving way, or talk to your friends to see what they think, about the possibility of you having Alzheimer's and the symptoms you're perceiving.

That being said, this chapter is going to overview some of the most commonly identifiable symptoms for Alzheimer's patients, to make it easier for you or a loved one to notice if Alzheimer's may be at work.

PLEASE get tested if you think you may have Alzheimer's – self diagnosis is not acceptable!!!

The symptom checklist for Alzheimer's:

- Does the person struggle with day to day tasks that used to be no problem for them?

- Is the person looking more tired lately?

- Is the person's attentiveness suffering, perhaps showing up in difficulty following a conversation or focus on a task?

- Is the person more confused, especially in places that don't make sense for that person to be confused?

- Do you find the person is often struggling to find the words to say?

- Is the person withdrawing socially from daily life and activities?

These behaviors are things that you can notice in friends, family, and often even in yourself. If you find you are answering yes to more than one or two of these questions, it may be time to seek out a medical opinion. Remember, even if it isn't Alzheimer's that's bothering your mind, it could be other things that still need to get checked out!

The Progression of Alzheimer's – Stages to Watch For

Alzheimer's, like any disease, goes through stages. This chapter will overview the typical stages of Alzheimer's so that you can better recognize them in yourself or your loved ones.

The formal stages/what's happening in the body
We'll get the formal stages out of the way first. You will not be able to recognize these stages, but they will help you to better understand what is happening to your loved one. Later, we will examine the informal stages – these are the ones you will most likely recognize.

Stage 1. Lesions
What it looks like?

- Lesions appearing and beginning to cause damage in the entorhinal cortex (in your head – not visible).

Things are not serious at this stage, and in fact you will not even be able to recognize outward symptoms yet – the brain damage is just beginning.

How long it lasts? This first stage has a long lifespan, and can last anywhere from 10 – 50 years before advancing.

Stage 2. Lasting damage to the hippocampus
What it looks like?

- The result of years of lesioning has caused brain damage at this point, specifically in the hippocampal region (a portion of the entorhinal cortex).
- Short term memory loss symptom begins to appear.

The hippocampus is responsible for memory, hence the appearance of the symptom visibly. This is where you may begin to see memory impairment, at least in short term items, and there may be personality changes in things like mood regulation (as the hippocampus also plays a role in this).

How long it lasts? This stage last between two and four years.

Stage 3. Spreading
What it looks like?

- The lesions that began in the entorhinal cortex are now spreading throughout the brain and impacting other areas.
- Symptoms apparent now.

As the damage spreads, the appearance of symptoms are increasing. Eventually Alzheimer's lesions will reach the areas of the brain you use to interpret familiarity, connect concepts, and to think about new ideas.

This is one of the most heartbreaking stages, as it's where the family is 'forgotten'.

How long this lasts? This stage lasts between two and eight years.

Stage 4. Moderate dementia
What it looks like?

- Muscle aches
- Bouts of irrational behaviour
- Paranoia

This stage sees the spread of the lesions and plaques to the frontal lobe of the brain, responsible for perception and sense of reasoning/ good judgement. This is why you see things like irrational behaviour, paranoia, or muscular aches, the brain is actually being messed with to create these symptoms.

People will absolutely have noticed by now, and the patient may even be misdiagnosed with dementia.

How long it lasts? This stage lasts between two and six years.

Stage 5. The final stages of Alzheimer's
What it looks like?

- Extreme dementia
- Inability to care for oneself
- Frequent health issues as a result of breakdowns of communication

How long it lasts? This stage typically lasts between two to four years.

This is the final stage of Alzheimer's, and unfortunately, as the name suggests, it typically only ends in death of the patient. By now, the patient will be unable to care for themselves at all, will be exhibiting irrational behaviour, will likely be at increased risk for health issues – and will be unable to communicate what the problems they are having internally are to obtain the proper medical care.

We will now take some time and consider the less formal symptoms of Alzheimer's, as you may find it hard to recognize 'brain damage', until it is far too late to help.

Informal Stages
Stage 1. Memory issues
What it looks like?

- Becoming forgetful of more than just daily tasks (car keys, what you were doing, etc.)
- Losing track of where you are
- Being frequently unable to recall names, places, etc.

This stage is often where misdiagnosis occurs. Some of the common things Alzheimer's is mistakenly diagnosed for include hormonal changes, or mental health issues that cause hormonal imbalances (like depression).

On the flip side of this, sometimes this stage is neglected or dismissed as "just getting older". The patient is still fully capable of communicating, even when they forget the word they're trying to reference. Understanding is fully intact, but recall is starting to slip here.

While the signs we listed above can be normal signs of typical memory lapses, increased frequency or severity of your forgetting can be a symptom, and should be checked out.

Stage 2. Where others start to worry
What it looks like?
- Repeating oneself repeatedly
- Breaking down communication into sentence fragments
- Some self awareness, potential for social embarrassment/ depression

This is where people begin to become concerned. You may be repeating yourself, or asking the same questions of people, or needing things explained differently because you just can't seem to get there.

Communication skills begin to break down here. This is because you're struggling now not just to remember the right word, but also to know what you're trying to say. You may find the person starts to speak in concepts, saying things like "where is the stuff we use to cover the leftovers" instead of "where is the plastic wrap".

This could also lead to social isolation, as implemented by the person suffering, to avoid the embarrassment of being seen as "crazy" or "senile". This is reflected in the fact that those around you will indeed begin to notice the changes in your behaviour, and may become concerned about them and express that concern.

That being said, this stage can go on for quite awhile before the person chooses to seek treatment, so watch for this, because the next stages are all a lot more severe.

Advanced Stages:

The stages upwards from two reflect an increasing tendency to forget, and – scariest of all – a lack of awareness of the difficulties others are seeing. This is where the Alzheimer's patient may frequently argue that they're "fine" to take care of themselves, when unfortunate caregivers have to battle them to seek treatment.

In the final stages of the disease, patients will no longer understand basic concepts (like night and day). They may revert to a time of comfort or happiness in the past, and think that it is several years ago. These changes effect the individual's ability to orient oneself (or find their way), and can result in many worrying nights for caregivers wondering if their loved one will find their way home. For the patient, it makes them largely unaware of what's going on. They can frequently find themselves in places they have no understanding or recollection of.

Finally, the person will likely be unable to communicate effectively. This can lead to a host of medical problems, because the person struggles to articulate even the most basic of information related to dehydration, or sources of infection, etc. As a result, unfortunately Alzheimer's all too often manages to kill with another health problem that the patient was unable to explain to their nurses.

This is where full supervision of the Alzheimer's patient becomes necessary, and it is a hard pill to swallow for many suffering from it. The advanced stages of Alzheimer's can result in depression, irritability, and other indicators that the person may sense they are not being treated like they used to – but they can't understand why.

When a person reaches the stages where they are unable to care for themselves and really struggling to communicate, the average life expectancy is 2.5 more years from that point. This is for a variety of reasons, and functions as an average.

Conclusions:

As you can see from our time lines, Alzheimer's is really a long lasting disease. The positive side of this is that your loved one can physically survive many years after a diagnosis, but of course, not without the lasting damage that living with Alzheimer's creates.

Potential Causes of Alzheimer's

Before we get into discussing what causes Alzheimer's, I want to be clear in saying that science is still unsure about this. Research has been going on for decades, but so far a lot of what we know to be the causes involve the physiological symptoms. Beyond the symptoms that cause the damage itself, all we know is that *something* is causing Alzheimer's.

So, physiologically speaking, what causes Alzheimer's? The neuron tangles that form, these tangles allow the buildup of plaque, which weakens and eventually damages connections in the brain.

What are some of the theories we have come up with to explain Alzheimer's? Let's take a look:

- Aluminum theory – In addition to the infamous tangles and plaque that characterize the brains of Alzheimer's sufferers, there is also a higher than normal amount of aluminum often found within. This has led some people to speculate that aluminum is related to getting Alzheimer's.

  This theory has even led some to change anti-antiperspirants, believing the aluminum content to be too high – and that it may build up over time.

- Mercury poisoning – Long term exposure to mercury could be one potential cause of Alzheimer's.

- Nutritional deficiencies (often Vitamins A & E, acetylcholine, or zinc are suspected) – We often look to the diet to see what causes our health problems, and Alzheimer's researchers are no exception. It is possible that a nutrient deficiency could be triggering the formation of a chemical that causes the tangles and plaque.

- Protein – Specifically, the Alzheimer's Disease Associated Protein (ADAP). This protein has been found after autopsy, but researchers speculate that if we could develop a way to identify it before death, perhaps we could do something about it if it is indeed the underlying cause.

- A virus – These things don't just infect your computers, researchers have speculated that Alzheimer's could actually be caused by a virus we don't yet know enough about.

Does Genetics Play A Role In Alzheimer's?

The chapter above overviewed some of the common neurological theories about what causes Alzheimer's, but what about genetics? For those of you who don't know, genetics is a term given to describe your genes, the bits of DNA you get from your parents at the time of conception.

DNA is like the blueprints for your body, it contains the 'plans' for everything from your eye color to your height, and it does often signify risk for health issues and other things.

Genetics play a role in the development of several health issues, and maybe even behavior problems, but do they play a role in Alzheimer's?

Researchers are very careful on what they say about this. Here, I will summarize the research findings, and then discuss the implications:

- People who suffer from Alzheimer's earlier in life tend to have abnormalities in chromosomes 1, 14, and 21.

- People who suffer from Alzheimer's later in life tend to have abnormalities in chromosome 19 and the creation of apoliprotein E (apoE).

- There is only a 10% hereditary correlation for Alzheimer's, meaning if someone in your family has Alzheimer's you are 10% more likely to get it.

These findings don't tell us a lot, but there are some things we can learn from them.

1) There's only a 10% hereditary link. This is very low, and suggests the influence of the environment is likely much stronger than the influence of your genes is on whether or not you will develop Alzheimer's.

2) Protein has been implicated in the development of Alzheimer's, though we do not yet understand how.

The truth is that research shows that environment and lifestyle choices must play a much larger role than family history for Alzheimer's, but that family history can play a role from time to time.

This guide will be going over some of the things you can do to reduce your risk, and what those risk factors are. Interestingly enough, nicotine is one of them! Nicotine has been known to help with memory, but damage other areas of the brain, changing the way a smoking Alzheimer's patient will experience Alzheimer's dramatically (initially for the better, but ultimately for the worse)!

Treating Alzheimer's

Alzheimer's is unfortunately currently classified as a disease without a cure. Science is constantly working to advance itself enough to being able to prevent Alzheimer's or completely banish it, but so far we are just finding symptoms of the problem and possible ways to treat those symptoms.

So, with treating the symptoms in mind, the medical profession proceeds to manage Alzheimer's as best as we can.

This chapter will overview some of the most common medical treatments for Alzheimer's. Later, we will talk about some of the natural things you can do, and some of the lifestyle choices you can make, but for right now we will discuss medication.

There are several medications that we use when trying to treat Alzheimer's, and we will review each of them. Rest assured, they have had success in prolonging individual's independence, and increasing quality of life. This is the good news.

Side Effects
The bad news is that these medications have side effects, and you should be aware of them. Estimates range, but current estimates are that as many as 20% of individuals taking Alzheimer's medications experience at least one significant side effect.

So what are some common side effects of taking medication?

- Aches
- Diarrhea
- Heartburn
- Increase in aggression – possibly because as you regain the understanding of what's going on around you, you become frustrated at the Alzheimer's disease entirely and take it out in your every day behaviour, but the point is that aggression is a potential side effect.
- Nausea, vomiting
- Other, rare side effects

We included the class "other, rare side effects" to reflect the fact that, occasionally, medications do cause differing effects on different people. We are all individuals, and the way our bodies process the medications has a lot to do with our bodily and behavioral response to those medications.

Extreme side effects

- Change in frequency and amount of urine
- Sudden seizure (particularly where seizures were not present before)
- Slowed pulse
- Jaundice in the eyes (yellowing)

Warning: If ANY of the symptoms above are present when you begin a medication, *let your health care professional know immediately!* You should not take risks with these symptoms, as they have been linked to more serious disorders and issues.

Seeking medical attention can stop a lot of nasty side effects in their tracks.

Medications

That being said, we're going to now go through the medications themselves. Feel free to use this chapter as a reference chapter, returning when you want more information.

Multiple Medication Possibility

Be aware that when treating Alzheimer's, people are seeking to treat a lot of symptoms. This can result in multiple medications, maybe some to deal with the Alzheimer's initial symptoms, and others to deal with the potential side effects of the drugs you're taking. The point is that you can end up with multiple prescriptions if being treated for Alzheimer's, so it's something to be aware of when feeling like one drug applies more than the others to your case.

Experimental Drugs?

What are they trying to do?

Since we can't really provide names (there's too many to list right now), we'll walk you through the purpose of the newest research of experimental Alzheimer's drugs. Alzheimer's experimental drugs are currently trying to stimulate the production of acetylcholine in the brain.

If you don't know what acetylcholine is, don't worry, it is a chemical in the brain that Alzheimer's basically takes away. By working to stimulate production of it, these drugs may be able to help stave off some of the damage of AD, and maybe even provide some recovery options.

These drugs will remain classified as experimental until the Food and Drug Administration (the FDA) approves them for public use. The bottom line is that researchers are looking to fight Alzheimer's in any way they can, and right now that looks a lot like focusing on treating the symptoms and slowing down the disease – while we search for a cure.

Only about 40% of patients actually see a reversal of the damage done to their brains, and the damage has to have been fairly recent for even that effect to take place. There is hope in medication, but there isn't a miracle. Keep that in mind when considering the goals of the medications, because they're here to make sure that you and your loved ones are comfortable and as happy as possible, and to give you as much time unaffected by Alzheimer's as is possible.

This is why this guide focuses on preventing Alzheimer's. Once you have Alzheimer's, there are things you can do to manage it, but you unfortunately cannot be as free as you would without having it at all. So many of our chapters offer advice that may seem unimportant right now, but could not be more critical in the war on Alzheimer's disease.

NonSteroidal Anti-Inflammatory Drugs (NSAIDs)

What are they?

These are your standard Advil, Aleve, Motrin, Tylenol, your over the counter pain relievers.

How are they used?

NSAIDs are best used in small dosages. Usually Alzheimer's patients wind up on 175mg-500mg or less per day, depending on the specific NSAID being used at the time.

Why do they work?

Studies have shown that NSAIDs have been associated with better performance on cognitive skill tests in Alzheimer's patients, significantly better performances than when taking no medication or when overdoing the NSAID dosage.

When taken properly, NSAIDs seem to help Alzheimer's patients hold on to a bit of cognitive capacity they may lose sooner otherwise.

What are the side effects?

The side effects of NSAIDs are relatively low key, primarily focusing on stomach irritation. The only danger to NSAIDs is prolonged usage, or overdoing the dosages, as this has been connected to stomach bleeding, kidney failure, and other nasty side effects.

When are they called in?

NSAIDs are a popular category of drug for treating Alzheimer's early symptoms. The reason for this is because they have had a lot of success with milder forms of damage present in the brain.

One particular study, done with mice, did see the reduction of beta amyloid, a component of the plaque that is so characteristic of Alzheimer's. It is believed that this component of the plaque may be related to the onset of damage. This is thought because the mice who were taking NSAIDs did not experience any increase in the amount of plaque.

That being said, NSAIDs do nothing to actually treat the brain damage being caused by Alzheimer's. The disease will still be progressing, NSAIDs have just been associated with delayed onset of the symptoms.

Prevention, Not Treatment

The unfortunate reality of Alzheimer's is that once you are diagnosed, you know what's ahead. Medications and treatments can work to delay its onset, but eventually the Alzheimer's will have damaged your brain to the point that you no longer understand basic concepts.

This is a terrifying idea, and I recognize that. Alzheimer's disease scares many people when they think of aging, and rightfully so. My point here is not to scare you, but to encourage you to reach out to your caregivers and go to the library together, pick up some guides on what's ahead and how to best understand it. We have made a list in the appendix following this guide to get you started.

That being said, the primary point of this guide is to share my research on how to prevent Alzheimer's. Whether you have Alzheimer's yourself, it runs in your family, or you just know someone else who has it, you should be looking to help protect yourself and those around you from its damaging effects.

Do not think that there is no hope if it does run in your family, remember the low rated link between family history and Alzheimer's. This guide is going to provide tips and tricks to improve your lifestyle choices and arm your body to fight off Alzheimer's.

Please note that even if you do have Alzheimer's, you can work to delay the onset of symptoms by following the tips in this book. Although you know where your mind will eventually go, you have no idea when it will get there.

For some, it is too late, but for you reading this right now – there are steps to be taken to protect yourself and your loved ones. Those steps involve getting and remaining mentally sharp, and no matter what you're thinking right now, you can do this!

There Are Natural Methods Too!

Alright, we're through with explanations. You've already read about what Alzheimer's is, what it does to the body, and the medications used to treat it. Now it's time to get into what you really are here for, the research on prevention.

Moving forward from this chapter on, I will focus this guide only on presenting the tried and true methods to prevent Alzheimer's. All of them center around the health of your brain, and the health of your body. By keeping your brain and body healthy, we will do everything to arm you with defences against Alzheimer's disease so that – even if you do eventually get it – you will see delay in its onset (at the very least) and probably no onset at all!

So what kind of methods are we going to look into?

Well, we will mention a few. First, I will mention the medications. There are two primary drugs used to delay Alzheimer's onset, and they are called Aricept and Cognac. Both of these drugs have been approved by the FDA, and are widely used as cholinesterase inhibitors.

You may be wondering what about acetylcholine. Recall, acetylcholine is the neurotransmitter we've been talking so much about. Well, what makes acetylcholine so important is its ability to inhibit cholinesterase when it's properly broken down. The drugs we have mentioned above focus on doing just that, and so will the treatments this guide lists.

The difference is that this guide will be helping you to see this breakdown of acetylcholine naturally.

I mention medications briefly and I mention them here because, although I do recognize you want to know the names of the medications, this guide is naturally based. I identified these medications to get at the root of what we are trying to do to delay and prevent Alzheimer's, and that is to inhibit cholinesterase currently.

I will be providing you with herbs, minerals, and vitamins that you need to be adding to your diet. I will show you things you can do to keep your mind sharp. I will even provide exercises that can help in the path to preventing Alzheimer's. But above all? I will educate you every single step of the way as to why I am doing these things and what makes them so important to you.

Do not rush out and grab up acetylcholine supplements just yet. Read through the following chapters. I will outline several herbs, minerals, and vitamins that all work to naturally supplement your bodies ability to do this. I will also explain every step of the way why these elements should be important to you, so that you will approach your diet with knowledge as well as willpower.

Lastly I would like to note how to best use this chapter. I have listed the treatments based on their classifications. For example, a lot of vitamins have *antioxidant* properties, so we'll talk about antioxidants. Strengthening your immune system is a great way to stay healthy, so we'll talk about the minerals that can do that. And so on. By breaking it down by category, I have made this guide easier for you to turn back to when you're struggling with specific elements in your diet.

For example, if you're struggling with free radical cells, you will want to go to the antioxidant section of this guide, whereas if you're weakened from infection already you may want to work on building your immune system.

The bottom line is that education is a huge tool in keeping your mind sharp, and the more you know about how to prevent Alzheimer's, the better off you will be in fighting it off. This guide is going to provide you with a lot of information, summarized in the easiest to understand ways possible, and in ways that allow you to refer back to chapters.

Come back and review the charts in the following pages at any time. I have laid them out to lay out your options, and there are several. Don't expect yourself to have them all memorized.

Ready? Let's go.

Antioxidants

What do they do?

To understand what antioxidants do for your health, you need to understand free radical cells. The human body is made up of millions and millions of cells, each of those cells are composed of atoms. I know, I know, but it's only a basic science lesson.

What you need to know is that there are some cells that do not care about the body, called free radical cells, and if they go unchallenged they will distribute themselves throughout the body – wreaking havoc wherever they go. This has a negative impact on the health of several bodily functions and organs, but what we're concerned with today is the impact on the brain. When free radicals hit the brain, they begin to damage neurons and weaken connections, connections your mind needs to effectively process incoming information.

This is what leads to things like memory loss, tremors, and ultimately the terrifying loss of the ability to connect even the most basic concepts.

As you may have guessed by now, antioxidants fight free radical cells. They specifically target them out before further damage can be caused.

Where do we get them?

You can get antioxidants from your diet. Several foods naturally contain antioxidants, but especially organic foods and whole grains.

You do also get some from your body itself, but if you don't supplement these natural levels as you age, you will find they aren't helping as much (because there just aren't as many of them as there used to be).

Alpha Lipoic Acid (ALA)

What does it do?

Alpha Lipoic Acid is a specific antioxidant. We've talked about antioxidants and their function just above, they battle free radical cells.

What distinguishes ALA from all of the rest is its ability to not only act as an antioxidant, but also stimulate the growth of other antioxidants, and it stimulates glutathione.

Glutathione helps to actually reverse the effects of nerve damage, and heighten the defence of cells all at once. Research has gotten excited about ALA for this reason, it stimulates glutathione (which can help reduce nerve damage) and also other antioxidants (only serving to double the effect you're getting).

Thanks to contemporary research, we now understand that ALA is amazing not only for its links with reversed nerve damage, but also for its potential link with improving memory. The scientists behind these studies are getting excited, and with good reason, ALA could well be the discovery of our day!

Where do you find it?

The body naturally produces alpha Lipoic acid, but not in quantities high enough to make a difference to your antioxidant levels. So where should you look to get more? The answer again is diet. ALA is primarily found in liver, spinach, and yeast.

Acetyl-L-Carnitine (ALC)

How is it used?

ALC is an antioxidant. We've already talked about this a lot, but antioxidants are great for preventing Alzheimer's – and for your health – because of the way they prevent the formation of free radical cells, and help your body to fight off existing ones.

On top of its antioxidant properties, ALC also stimulates acetylcholine within the brain. Acetylcholine is that neurotransmitter that Alzheimer's attacks, and any supplement that increases its supply should be considered extremely valuable in the battle to prevent and delay Alzheimer's. ALC does just that by maintaining healthy acetylcholine quantities in the brain.

ALC is also used internationally to treat neural disorders because of its ability to help reverse brain damage. This is likely a function of its abilities to stimulate acetylcholine, but regardless, we know it works.

One clinical study examined over 500 Alzheimer's and dementia patients and found that ALC was able to help reverse some of the brain damage that occurred, and to inhibit memory deterioration. Interestingly, it also helped improve communication abilities and concentration levels in the clinical study.

Where do you get it?

ALC does naturally occur within the body but, like so many other things, it slows down production as we get older. Thus we recommend getting ALC in supplementary form, in 1000-1200mg/ daily dosages.

Boron – And How to Use It Safely

What it does?

Boron is a mineral that has been linked with improved memory function, increased strength, and muscular function improvement.

Where to get it and how to be safe with it?

If you know much about boron, you may already know that it was outlawed in the 1950s. The reason for this is that boron was being used as a preservative at the time, and though it does have preserving qualities, it was being used in such high quantities that it made itself toxic.

The body can handle boron, but only in extremely low dosages (3mg/daily should be considered a maximum). That being said, you do not need any boron supplements, just to indulge in some whole grains, some leafy veggies, or fruits (apples, grapes, pears, etc.). So you can get it perfectly safely as long as you only obtain it through diet!!!

Curry

This spice probably doesn't take a lot to recognize. It is a staple of Indian cooking. Something else interesting about India? Its residents are four times less likely to end up having Alzheimer's than their North American counterparts.

How does it work?
Curry contains curcumin, a completely natural food preservative and food dye. Curcumin has also been associated with anti-inflammatory properties, antioxidant properties, and protein inhibition.

The protein inhibition function is especially interesting to people who are trying to prevent Alzheimer's, as it stops some of the plaque (and thus can either delay onset or prevent onset of Alzheimer's).

Where do you get it?
Curry is easy to obtain, spice up some of your diet with it regularly and you'll be well on your way to preventing Alzheimer's! Hit up your local grocery store for the spice.

Ginkgo Biloba

What does it do?

Ginkgo biloba is a herb with many talents. It has been used for ages as an herbal aid for memory problems, it has been known to improve circulation, and it acts as an antioxidant as well.

Western science is beginning to pick up on the importance of this Ancient Asian herbal remedy, and we're starting to see some tremendous potential results.

Ginkgo biloba has been associated with repairing brain damage, though mainstream medicine has not yet accepted this fact, and unanimously has been hailed for its ability to improve blood flow to the brain. The important thing you need to know about blood flow to the brain? More nutrients and healthy cells getting to the brain to impact the plaques and tangles that are forming.

These are just some of the health benefits of this truly powerful Asian herb. This little herb effects you just as a drug would. Now that being said, do not take supplements of ginkgo biloba if you struggle with blood issues.

Where do you find it?

You primarily find Ginkgo biloba at the health food store, but you should not start it without a professional medical consultation. The reason for this is that ginkgo biloba does thin the blood, and for some people this can cause problems more so than others. Seek medical advice if you are considering taking Ginkgo biloba, and only ever stick to a low dosage of under 200mg/day.

Huperzia Serrata (Huperzine)

What does it do?

Huperzine has been used for generations by Chinese herbalists. It has been hailed as a cure for fever, and an anti-inflammatory, but we care about it because of its ability to work with memory loss. Huperzine works with acetylcholine in such a way that it actually mimics the most popular drugs out there that we've talked about.

It should be used extensively during the early stages of Alzheimer's, as it has the potential to improve memory, but that function is something everyone can use a bit more of. So even if you don't have Alzheimer's, you can take huperzine.

Where do you get it?

There are several places you can get huperzine from, some tasty and some not so great. I recommend using qian ceng ta (a Chinese herb). In contrast to this, club moss works, but doesn't tend to taste good.

Be forewarned again that dosage comes into play here. 50 mcg/ twice per day (MICROGRAMS not milligrams) is a safe dosage, but 30 is the recommended dosage.

Exceeding recommended dosages can lead to severe side effects such as diarrhea, headache, nausea, muscle cramps, and vomiting.

Consult a medical professional if you are thinking of taking huperzine to be sure it does not conflict with your prescriptions for Alzheimer's already.

Lecithin

The short answer to this question is that lecithin provides choline to the body. Choline, as we've talked about, acts as an aid to the body in a lot of different ways. The long answer to lecithin benefits is that there are several: from lowering cholesterol to potentially improving memory.

In terms of how lecithin is used in lowering cholesterol, lecithin stimulates the metabolism. Your body's metabolism is what breaks down foods into fat and other nutrients, lecithin stimulates this process to move quicker while working to improve cell walls – to decrease the chance of fatty bits of cholesterol clinging on.

In terms of how it may improve memory, lecithin has showed some evidence in animal studies of being able to improve nerve impulse transmissions, which helps in memory. This finding is debated, but what is known for sure is that it does help protectively coat the brain – so it does help the brain no matter what.

The final important function of lecithin is in its ability to help the body absorb other minerals. This means that anything you take after lecithin will be better absorbed than if you had taken none at all, and works to bolster your efforts at changing your diet.

Where you get it?
Lecithin is often found either in capsules or in your diet. Some types of foods that include lecithin are egg yolks, fish, grains, legumes, and yeast.

Vitamins C & E

Why do we talk about them together?

Vitamins C and E get talked about a lot, and most often in conjunction with one another. The reason for this is their complementary functions. Vitamin C tends to pave the way for vitamin E (and other vitamins and minerals) to get their work done more effectively, by strengthening your immune system. This has a lot to do with the effects that it has.

What do they do?

Vitamin C builds the immune system's line of defences by supplementing other antioxidant minerals and vitamins in their effectiveness. This is why we so often see it paired off with other vitamins, because it enables them to not just do their job but to do it better by promoting antioxidant properties in all (and thus resulting in a lot less free radicals damaging your body).

Vitamin C also has been associated with battling high cholesterol (specifically atherosclerosis). In atherosclerosis, the artery walls can be damaged, but with Vitamin C the walls are already strengthened – saving your arteries a lot of damage that could otherwise occur.

Vitamin E on the other hand, acts as an antioxidant. This means that as we talked about above, it fights free radicals. However, vitamin E also prevents fat from oxidizing, preventing the formation of future free radicals and also improving cholesterol levels.

These vitamins work hand in hand to strengthen your immune system and fight off free radicals, and help your cholesterol to boot!

Where do you get these vitamins?

First, we want to make a final note about the importance of taking these vitamins together. They help each other out functionally, so make sure that if you are going to take a supplement it contains both.

That being said, the natural place to get vitamins C and E are in whole foods or whole food supplements. Whole foods and whole food supplements focus on providing multiple vitamins in one sitting. This gives your body more tools to work with, and helps greatly not just with battling Alzheimer's, but also with battling other health conditions because of the way that the vitamins complement each other.

Keep this in mind when considering vitamins C & E – take them together, and get them from whole foods or whole food supplements!

Zinc

What does it do?

Zinc inhibits plaque build up. You can already see then why it's immensely helpful for Alzheimer's patients. Alzheimer's patients often suffer from deficiencies in zinc additionally, meriting enough interest to suggest that getting zinc may help them.

Zinc also has other health benefits, such as to your cholesterol, because of its ability to prevent plaque formation. Conversely, having a deficiency in zinc can lead to health problems.

Where do you get it from?

Your diet will be your primary source of your zinc, specifically fish, meats, poultry, and even soy products. You can also find it in fenugreek, a herb that contains zinc.

Now, when considering supplementing your zinc levels, you must also take into account your copper levels. There is approximately a 10% balance of copper to zinc, so if you're taking 50mg of zinc you have also added 5mg of copper to your diet. Be aware of this, and moderate. You should only really be taking 50mg/daily of zinc, and never more than 100.

General Health of Your Brain and Body

Now, everything we've discussed so far in terms of preventing Alzheimer's has been discussed in terms of herbs, minerals, and vitamins that specifically have benefits for patients with Alzheimer's/ aspects of Alzheimer's.

The truth is that you can also prevent Alzheimer's by working to keep your body and brain healthy in general, so the next selection of herbs, minerals, and vitamins will relate to the general health of your body and brain. Don't worry, we'll still stop each step of the way to explain what's important and why.

Omega 3 Fatty Acids

What's so great about omega 3s?

Omega 3 fatty acids are wonderful for a lot of reasons related to your health, not the least of which is how they help you to reduce your levels of mercury (see later chapters for why you should be concerned about this).

Where do you get them?

Omega 3s are found naturally in eggs, but can also be taken in supplement form. *If you are taking supplements, please read the label.* We cannot say it enough, manufacturers often cut corners that only lead to damaging your health if you don't pay attention.

In terms of omega 3 supplements, the unfortunate reality is that the 'corner cut' is often higher levels of mercury. Get your pills analyzed before you take them, read reviews, and pay attention to those labels to avoid counteracting the positive impact the omega 3 supplements should be having.

Vitamin B Family

What's so great about Vitamin B?

Vitamins from the B family (especially the all powerful B6 and B12) work to improve brain functioning, mental state (often used in the treatment of depression), and improving the health of your blood.

In terms of how these vitamins help, vitamin B12 breaks down homocysteine, an amino acid that increases the 'bad cholesterol' (Low Density Lipoprotein/LDL). When vitamin B12 and folic acid are taken together, your bad cholesterol decreases dramatically, to give you a healthier you.

Individuals who have Alzheimer's are often deficient in vitamins in the B family, so it may be worth taking a supplement to see if it helps improve your symptoms. Speak to a medical professional if you are suffering from depression or Alzheimer's though before engaging in treatment yourself, as we have stated numerous times, you want to stay within the healthy range of dosages.

Where do you get it from?

People can often get all of the vitamin B they need from eggs, fruits, and leafy veggies. If you're still struggling or think you may be deficient, you can take a multivitamin, and in extreme cases vitamin B can be taken by injection.

Why Worry About The Brain Anyway?

So for all this talk about trying to eat the right things to keep yourself healthy and happy, I wanted to take a minute to explain to you why these things are so important.

First of all, a healthy diet has been linked time and time again to lower levels of stress, less instances of illness, and higher levels of happiness. If that's not enough for you, it's also linked to your health! This may seem obvious, but consider this: if you were eating as you should be right now you should have only very limited issues with blood pressure, low-cholesterol levels, and an immune system capable of fighting off a lot more than a weakened one!

Additionally, eating healthy provides your brain with the nutrients that it needs to promote your mental health, preventing chemical imbalances and, yes, Alzheimer's.

Keep in mind too, that eating healthy doesn't have to be terribly hard. There are several delicious foods that are good for you, and that can provide multiple vitamins and minerals all at once.

The best foods to work into your diet? Leafy veggies and whole grains. These two food groups cover almost all of the vitamins and minerals necessary in the battle to keep your brain healthy.

Also, fiber! Fiber is a great source of a lot of health benefits, and can also be found in leafy veggies and whole grains!

Getting your nutrients straight from your diet is the best way to naturally present Alzheimer's. That's why I have spent so much time on it in this book, I believe it's the key to helping you lead a healthier lifestyle and staying mentally fit.

That being said, if you're struggling to make your diet cover all of your nutritional needs, consider herbal teas or supplements. These supplements can be just as effective at providing the nutrients, and if you read the labels to watch out for additives, can also be almost as natural. Many herbs can be made into tea, added to salad, or even just used to spice up a meal.

What You DON'T Want In Your body

We've spent a lot of time talking about what to put in your body for a happier and healthier you and how these substances can set you on the path to avoid Alzheimer's, but what we haven't looked at yet is some things you may want to avoid.

In terms of diet, let's take a moment and discuss processed food. Processed food may seem like it's the more convenient option, but think about the ways in which you're poisoning yourself with it. Processed foods often contain aluminum, mercury, and other toxic substances to your body. It's a big sacrifice for a little convenience, don't you think?

That being said, diet is not the only thing you want to avoid.

There are two primary substances that are worth discussing here, aluminum and mercury. While science is unclear as to how they interact fully with Alzheimer's, it is clear that there is something going on between Alzheimer's patients and these chemicals.

For this reason, a lot of people want to know how to reduce the levels of these chemicals in their daily lives. We'd like to show you how, so please consider the following chapter a mini-guide.

Aluminum

*What's **NOT** so great about aluminum?*
We have already discussed aluminum as part of the potential causes of Alzheimer's, so you probably can already guess what's not so great about it. People who struggle with Alzheimer's often have higher levels of aluminum in their system than people who do not.

For that reason, we're going to take some time here and dedicate it to letting you know how to control your aluminum levels. We will mention as a disclaimer here that the medical community is not at all certain that aluminum is a cause of Alzheimer's, it's just a part of a theory right now.

Where do you get it from?
Your body does naturally produce a certain level of aluminum, and though we don't know why it's there, there isn't much you can do about that. However, did you know that tap water contains aluminum? How about antiperspirants? Both of these substances can have you raising your levels without thinking about it. Dialysis too is a medical treatment that raises your levels of aluminum.

How do you control it?
So, what do you do? You can work to lower your bodily levels of aluminum by taking a combination of 800-1200 mg of malic acid and 200-400 mg of magnesium. These substances work together, the acid working to break down aluminum within the system while the magnesium prevents it from being re-absorbed into the body. These two chemicals are great ways to cleanse your bodily levels of aluminum.

Mercury

What's NOT so great about Mercury?

Mercury is another substance that seems to have a mysterious interaction with Alzheimer's. Although not as much is understood about mercury as is about the aluminum connection, many people seek to reduce their mercury intake in their day-to-day lives when trying to live healthier.

Where do you get it from?

Mercury is found in two primary sources: fish and fillings. Now, we're not going to suggest that you avoid all fish, because mercury is not normally present in them, but there are polluted fish that can raise your bodily levels of mercury.

Similarly, fillings. We aren't going to say don't get any fillings, but to watch how often you get metal fillings (amalgam), which tend to be associated with higher levels of mercury.

How do you control it?

In terms of your diet, you can control your intake of mercury by eating only fish that you know where they've been (so only wild fish), and avoiding canned tuna. This reduces the likelihood of getting polluted fish, and thus contributes to lower mercury levels.

In terms of the dentist, while you can't tell someone necessarily how to do his/her job, you can request resin fillings. More and more dental offices are shifting toward resin fillings (as they tend to look better) already, so you may not need to worry about this, just try to avoid the metal ones when possible. You can also consider requesting that your old fillings be replaced if you are really concerned or have a high amount of metal fillings.

Alcohol and Nicotine – The Bad Guys in Most Health Food Guides

It shouldn't come as any big surprise that in a guide discussing how to be healthy and happy, I recommend you avoid alcohol and smoking. Let's talk about why.

Okay, so smoking is bad for you. Go figure. But did you know that research actually initially seemed to show that smoking could contribute to the *prevention* of Alzheimer's?! Crazy right? But nicotine has certain death delaying properties for cells, which temporarily put off the onset of the disease. The problem comes with the fact that cigarettes are not only (or even mostly) composed of nicotine. There are several other harmful substances contained within cigarettes that are why I recommend absolutely avoiding them.

Smoking has been linked with heart disease, with strokes, and poor blood flow. You've probably seen the pictures of what it does to your lungs, so just do yourself a favour and avoid it – your body will thank you.

Now let's move on to alcohol. Researchers have long been divided on whether the potential benefits outweigh the risks of indulging in a little bit of wine here or there.

Some of the research has indeed shown that *small* drinks every now and then have been linked with the reduction of risk for heart disease and stroke. Alcohol thins the blood a bit, allowing good cholesterol (high density lipoprotein/HDL) to flow easier, and making it harder for LDL (bad cholesterol) to build up. These things may sound good, but it's all hinged on the term "moderate" consumption of alcohol.

The problem then becomes that most people do not have "small drinks". We as a society tend to binge when we do drink. So I have presented the research above as a caution. It's your decision whether to drink or not, just ensure that if you do it is only small amounts "here and there", not a daily occurrence.

The research has been presented to you. This is why smoking and alcohol are bad for you, and these are the areas where they can potentially assist. The decision is now in your hands as to whether or not you think it's worth it to indulge.

I will say that in terms of preventing Alzheimer's, neither smoking nor alcohol seems to help. Nicotine arguably can, but not in cigarette form and only small amounts of drinking are beneficial to your health.

The choice is yours.

High Cholesterol

What's a chapter on cholesterol doing in a book about preventing Alzheimer's? Let's take a look at what cholesterol actually is and then see if you can take a wild guess.

Cholesterol itself is not a bad thing. It is a necessary part of every single cell within your body, as it protectively coats the all important cell membrane. This is the "good" function of cholesterol. The "bad" function of cholesterol is to attach to the cell and cause little blockages that make it harder for your blood to pass through. This causes higher blood pressure, poor circulation, and ultimately damages your arteries.

Arteriosclerosis is a condition where cholesterol has built up to the extent that the artery walls have thickened, and is one potential result of high cholesterol. Another potential result is heart attack or stroke, as it's been made more difficult for your blood to get through.

So how does this relate to Alzheimer's? In two very distinct ways that we will cover in the following discussions. There is definitely a connection, but it can be complex, so bear with me as I try to explain.

Amyloid-beta proteins
As we know, Alzheimer's hallmark is the neuron tangles and the buildup of amyloid plaque. So what do these plaques have to do with cholesterol?

Amyloid beta proteins are normally involved with cholesterol regulation, but when cholesterol gets out of control, they try to fight back by producing more of these proteins. This process, while good in intention, ultimately leaves extra amyloid beta proteins laying around to be used in the buildup of this plaque.

Especially because we so strongly suspect that the plaque is related to the progression of the disease, you can really see here where high cholesterol is connected to Alzheimer's.

Homocysteine

Amino acids are another key component to your body, always breaking down and rebuilding into other amino acids. When methionine breaks down, attempting to help the body to break down fat, homocysteine results.

Homocysteine is normally present in the range of 5-15 micromoles in the average person. In a person with Alzheimer's however, this range is much closer to 20 and above micromoles. This elevation reflects itself in difficulties with the methylation process, leading to brain damage and differing levels of neurotransmitters.

This is yet another connection we've been able to make where we're unsure which causes which, but we are paying attention.

The body does naturally protect against homocysteine, to an extent, in the form of estrogen. Estrogen prevents homocysteine levels from getting out of control, while it is being produced within the body. Please note that after menopause, or if you are male, this could mean you are already lacking and need to consider supplementing your estrogen levels or finding another way to control homocysteine.

So what do I recommend? Seek a medical professional's attention and get your homocysteine levels checked. These are not always looked for on a typical blood test, but can be checked at your request. Pay particular attention to this/get it done urgently if your family has a history of heart disease.

Finding your levels of homocysteine are out of the normal range? Consider your folic acid/Vitamin B levels. This is a vitamin that can be taken from multivitamins or prenatal vitamins (as it has been linked with the prevention of spina bifida as well). If you're not getting enough, you can supplement your diet by taking a 400MICROgram supplement. This acid helps to regulate your homocysteine levels.

Conclusions

Cholesterol should be managed. It has a good function for your body, the issue with it only comes when you let your cholesterol get out of control. Higher cholesterol levels have been linked with both amyloid beta protein and homocysteine production, both of which naturally lend themselves to the damage Alzheimer's works to wreak in your body.

It is worth noting that cholesterol is bad for your health completely separate of Alzheimer's as well. You are risking heart attack, stroke, and brain damage when you let your cholesterol skyrocket.

Your family history can impact your cholesterol levels, as can your diet. While you can't control your genetics, you can begin to adjust your diet to a lower fat and lower cholesterol diet, thus promoting healthy cholesterol levels.

Already have bad cholesterol? Don't worry, you can correct it in as little as two months with the proper dietary considerations.

All of that being said, you must be aware by now that I like to keep you informed of both sides of a research equation, and to that end, the next chapter reviews differing potential evidence about high cholesterol!

Research Controversy about High Cholesterol

I want to be as clear as possible, high cholesterol has been linked with a host of bad health effects. However, recently some controversial research has emerged about the potential *benefits* of high cholesterol.

You read that right. On May 24, 2005, research was documented within the Neurology publication that linked high cholesterol and some level of dementia prevention in older people. The age was key here, as older people seemed to be the ones who benefited from this effect. What this study ended up doing was muddying the waters.

What we know is this: cholesterol does do some good things for the cell (see our note on the 'good function' of cholesterol). This is critical especially as we age, because our cells are breaking down faster than the body can produce in some cases. However, high cholesterol diets have been linked with health problems.

The idea that's being raised to you to consider is, do older people not need to worry about their cholesterol? Is it potentially good for them to not worry about it? Or is there something else going on here?

Researchers will continue to question these links. The majority of research does urge you to control your cholesterol, this research may just suggest the addition of the phrase "control it when you're younger".

So now you know the controversy.

Controlling Your Cholesterol Levels – Should you be On a Statin drug?

Research published in May, 2005 looked at around 70 patients and linked the use of statin drugs with progressively improved cognitive function. So what do Statin drugs do? They're used to target cholesterol.

Pharmaceutical manufacturers cheered, Lipitor, Crestor, and Zocor profited. Nobody seemed to want to recognize that it may be the lowered cholesterol that's linked to improved cognitive function, not the presence of the drug itself.

They also didn't want to talk about the side effects. Statin drugs have been known to cause anything from muscle soreness to, in extreme cases, acute kidney failure, and everything like nausea in between.

What my point is here is that although Statin drugs do help with the prevention of Alzheimer's, they may do so by lowering your cholesterol – something you could do naturally anyway.

Does Meat Contribute To Alzheimer's?

In the 1990s a small string of controversial research emerged relating to Alzheimer's. Specifically, researchers claimed to have found a link between developing Alzheimer's and eating certain meats, and the prion disease was implicated.

Prion disease effects the brain, and does so by forming plaques. Forming plaques as you know is a precursor to Alzheimer's. We have known this for awhile, but what was now up for debate was whether or not we could be finding prion disease in some of our meat. This relates to methods of disease contraction, and is still hotly debated.

Current research suggests that it could be possible that meat is transferring the prion disease. The reason for this is that prion primarily affects the brain, and prion does not have DNA or a signature to look for. This means that even the most effective meat packaging plant does not stand much of a chance of figuring out if their meat is carrying the prion disease.

To support this assumption that meat is associated with Alzheimer's, we can look to India. India has the lowest instance of Alzheimer's globally, and India also has a law against killing cows, or gaining access to beef. When we compare India's 1-1.4 cases per 100 people to the US and Europe's 3.1-8.7 per 100 people, it does make it seem as though there may be a connection.

Dr. Murray Waldman describes these effects in his book Dying for a Hamburger. It covers prion disease, mad cow disease, Creutzfeldt-Jakob disease, and goes through how these germs are easier to transfer through meat.

The truth is that these findings are still controversial, and largely based on seemingly circumstantial evidence, but they are something you can consider if you'd like when altering your diet to prevent Alzheimer's.

The Importance of Eating Organic

Organic food are those foods that have been grown in a pesticide, and herbicide free environment, in other words, as naturally as possible.

(For meats this works out to being animals butchered without the use of growth hormones, and have not been confined to inhumane spaces).

Organic food has been gaining popularity for the last 10 years at least. Researchers are finding time and time again that organic food just how good organic food is for you, and have linked it to several health and personal benefits.

Free range chicken eggs for example have been known to contain fewer hormones than those which were not raised free range. This may produce a higher yield for the farmer in question, but does not make hormones good for human beings to indulge in in their daily diet.

Another added benefit of organic foods is the things that are present in them (that are not in their pesticide sprayed counterparts). An example of this is flavonoids. Flavonoids are a naturally occurring part of fruits and vegetables. They take care of the plant (banishing bugs and fighting off germs), and also prevent the spread of free radicals – making them an antioxidant. These flavonoids are a fantastic part of what makes eating fruits and vegetables such a great idea, but in fruits and vegetables that were sprayed with pesticides these flavonoids do not occur in nearly so high a quantity.

In other words? You lose out on the benefits of the food you're eating if it is not organically grown.

Recall that earlier we touched on the fact that antioxidants help you to prevent Alzheimer's, and consider the implication. Organic food is significantly better for preventing Alzheimer's than non organic foods, no matter what the cost.

Supermarkets have been working to lower the cost of organic foods to make them available to more and more consumers. The price gap between organic and non organic foods is lower than ever before, but if you're still struggling to afford organic, you can always make the shift towards canned goods, or hit up your local farmer's market, as these are usually cost effective sources of organically grown fruits and vegetables.

However you plan on getting it, make sure that organic foods are an aspect of the way that you plan your diet.

The Importance of Education

As your parents probably told you, education is a huge part of life. Whether you have it or you don't, it's taking an effect on you.

Working to obtain an education has been associated with higher incomes, a reportedly happier lifestyle, and more career opportunities. This may or may not be news to you, but consider the following:

People who *don't* work to obtain an education increase their risk for health issues and, indeed, dementia. In fact, those who have only an 8th grade education are twice as likely as those who went further to develop issues with cognitive impairment!

Researchers do not entirely understand this link, but estimate that it may have to do with the way that learning effects the brain. You see, as we go through life, we actually change our brain chemistry. We strengthen some connections between our neurons (pieces of material our brain is made up of), and we weaken others. We begin to specialize in certain areas, and our brain reflects that.

When you learn you 'work out' the neural connections in your mind, and when you 'exercise' those connections regularly, you increase your ability to stay (mentally) sharper, for longer periods of time than when you remain intellectually inactive. This is just as big a caution as the one against being physically inactive, you must stay mentally active.

So, how do you do this? No you don't have to go and get a university degree because you're afraid of Alzheimer's. Education is one way to stimulate your mind, but it's not the only way. Another way is by continually challenging your mind by learning new skills, languages, and even hobbies.

Studying in a school can be a great way to keep yourself mentally challenged on a constant basis, but you can do it even by working on new skills or trying one of the other activities listed above. The key is to keep your mind active for as long as possible and, much like with our body, this involves 'working out'!

Consider the following chapter on exercising your brain for more tips.

How to Work Out Your Brain

So we've been discussing how your brain needs to be worked out, much like the body, but you're probably wondering how.

Everyday experiences are constantly altering your mind, but it's important to make sure to choose at least some of these experiences selectively – with the intention of working out your brain. Just like the body needs more than 5 minutes of walking from your house to your car, your brain needs to be exercised more than just deciding what to wear and your regular patterns of thought throughout the day to work at its best.

You don't have to work to keep your brain functioning at its highest, and the truth is you may not feel the after effects for many years, but when you do you will regret your inactivity. An inactive brain is an unhappy brain, and it will show this by weakening different connections your mind is used to having.

So how do you do this? There are several methods, some of which we will now consider:

- Reading – The benefits of reading is that it really engages your mind. Try picking up a newspaper instead of turning on the TV. Listen to a book on your daily commute rather than numbing yourself. Force your brain to work on information a bit more frequently than it currently does.

- Eating Right – That's right, those dietary tips we gave you above benefit your brain too. By making sure you're eating right, you're providing your brain with resources (in the form of nutrients), and ensuring that you're well equipped to start any one of these working your brain out options.

The benefits of focusing on eating right are numerous: from health benefits to a better physique to ease of blood flow, your body and your mind will thank you for working on your diet. In addition, you'll be preventing obesity – a condition which increases the risk of dementia by over 74%!

- Exercising – A study published in 2003 in the New England Journal of Medicine stated findings of researchers that, when 124 participants were taken into account, people were significantly less likely to develop Alzheimer's when they regularly exercised. Exercising releases certain chemicals in the body that can be good for the brain too.

- Formal Education – We've talked about this, but the benefits of education can hardly be stressed enough. If you are interested in pursuing formal education, you will already be a long way to working out your brain.

- Logic Games – Chess, logical puzzles, even dancing. All of these activities stimulate your mind by requiring planning, reading, and thought. This is a great – and very fun – way to work out your brain!

- Puzzles – Much like reading, puzzles engage the mind by forcing you to reason and rationalize about where each piece will go.

Your brain can handle a lot, but you really have to push it to keep it working at its full capacity. By aiming to challenge yourself on a regular basis, you'll be a long way to strengthening your mind as well as your body, and yes you will be working towards preventing Alzheimer's.

The Importance of Exercise

Much like our chapter on alcohol and smoking, this chapter may seem like it's a bit obvious – exercising is good for you! However, there's a lot you likely don't know about the benefits of exercise, that I think are important motivators when you just don't want to get up and work out yet.

Benefits of Regular Exercise
- Better blood flow and general health of the circulatory system and ideal levels of nitric oxide.

- More efficient metabolic processing, particularly showing in the production levels of oxygen and glucose

- Better level of retention for memories.
  In one study, rats that exercised once improved their memory for at least three days following the session, and saw benefits within the brain for the following four weeks!

- Higher levels of antioxidants within the body, preventing additional free radical cells

- Lower cholesterol

- Lower levels of stress, and more efficient physical response to stress

- Longer retention of cognitive abilities, beyond age 70

You probably already know how great physical exercise is for your blood pressure and heart health overall, but did you know that it has been linked with the prevention of both Alzheimer's and dementia?

This link is thought to be a reflection of the circulatory system, as patients with Alzheimer's tend to struggle with circulation. Because exercising targets this system so early on, it has been linked with preventing Alzheimer's, all while keeping your blood pressure down and getting a handle on your cholesterol!

Good circulation is vital for a stable system, and is promoted best by cardiovascular exercising. It's also good for keeping your mind active and in shape, as the mind seems willing to follow the trends that the body sets.

What kind of exercise should you be doing?
We've already mentioned that aerobics are one great way to get your weekly workout sessions in, but there are other forms, specifically strength exercises and toning exercises.

Strength exercising, as the name implies, is focused on building strength through things like weight lifting, chin-ups, or push-ups. Toning exercises are similar, but also include things like squats and sit ups. These exercises will work to improve your health, your physique, and will even increase bone density, helping you to be a much healthier person just by working out.

Don't think that just because I'm recommending you exercise I'm going to tell you need to spend thousands of dollars on equipment or gym memberships. You can use a lot of things you commonly find around the home to do exercises, and that's only when you need supplies – often your own body is sufficient equipment to keep you in peak physical condition.

How often should you be exercising?

In terms of how much exercise you need to reap these benefits, experts tend to agree that working out at least three times per week (in 20-30 minute sessions) seems to be the best goal. It's worth noting that this "working out" should be heart pumping, heavy breathing exercise (aerobics work great), though it can be done in many forms and still see you being healthier and happier.

Fun fact: exercise is also associated with the release of endorphins, a neurotransmitter associated with happiness and overall well being! So you literally will be happier, just by working your body towards a healthier you!

Consulting a medical professional

Before undertaking a new spin class however, do take your current health into consideration. If you know that you're already extremely out of shape, head to the doctors for a physical and consult them about your workout routine. While exercising regularly is healthy, picking a routine that will push your system too hard is quite the opposite.

Stress Reduction

Stress can be good for your body, but only in the short term. Keeping yourself stressed out for long periods of time is bad for both your brain and your body, and thus stress reduction goes a long way in preventing things like dementia.

In fact, the Alzheimer's Prevention Foundation International and the Amen Clinic at the University of California have studied the effects of Kirtan/Kriya, and found that just doing the basic chants involved for 5 minutes resulted in significant changes in the brain. These changes activated the frontal lobes, most associated with reasoning and concentration.

By activating these areas, you are "working out your brain" - just by using an effective stress reduction method that's good for you anyway!

These findings have been supported repeatedly, by research done by scientists at Massachusetts General Hospital, Massachusetts Institute of Technology, Harvard, and Yale! These studies have also linked meditation with a higher quantity of grey brain matter, another sign of good brain health.

Things you can do to reduce stress and work out your brain:
- Kirtan/Kriya chants:
  Sa Ta Na Ma Ahh (2 minutes at a time)

- Completing word puzzles regularly

- Taking up puzzling as a hobby

- Take classes just to learn about something you've always wanted to

- Play with your memory, memorizing lyrics or telephone numbers

- Do math in your head

Conclusions

If you work with the brain, you get to keep yourself brain healthier for longer. If you don't, you don't. The choice is once again yours, and it can be tough with all of the mindless but fun activities out there.

Just keep in mind your brain needs exercise just like your body does, and you should be well on your way to a healthier mind, and a happier you!

Summary of Alzheimer's Prevention Tips

If you've made it this far, you've truly empowered yourself. You've armed yourself with a lot of knowledge. But realizing how much knowledge it is, you may be wondering how you're going to keep track of all this information.

Fear not, I have provided a summary chapter for you. Please feel free to print this, use it as a reference guide – returning when making a new plan to prevent Alzheimer's or to check how you've been progressing.

Eating Right

- Aim to eat well, and support that aim by making specific meal plans that ensure that you are getting all the nutrients your body needs.

- Focus your diet on organically grown fruits and vegetables, particularly green and leafy veggies. Remember that you want a diet high in antioxidants, vitamin B, and lecithin, as well as other healthy nutrient rich foods.

- Avoid processed foods. These are junk, they provide you with nothing and your body with only fat cells at best.

- Drink 8 glasses of water each day to ensure that you're staying hydrated. Being well hydrated has been associated with a host of medical and health benefits, but what you need to know right now is that it will improve your circulation and it will help your body to cleanse itself of waste.

- Take supplements where necessary. Some you may want to consider should be omega 3 fatty acids, folic acids, hyperzine, and any you are particularly deficient in. Consult a medical professional before beginning a supplement though!

Staying Physically Active

- Schedule a physical with your family doctor to get a read as to where you currently are in terms of cholesterol and physical fitness.

- Make sure you're being as active as you can, aiming to workout 3-5 times per week in 20-30 minute sessions.

  Physical fitness may reduce your risk of developing Alzheimer's by as much as 50%, and that doesn't even account for the host of other health benefits that regularly exercising affords you (like happiness, physique benefits, and more).

Staying Mentally Active

- Remember that your brain needs working out too, use it or lose it!

- Read, read, and read. Especially when you replace television time with reading, you're doing yourself a favor.

- Take up puzzling

- Play more logic games, like chess, checkers, crosswords, and word puzzles.

- Make a lifelong learner of yourself. Always try to be learning something new, play with your memory by trying to memorize simple things.

- Make an effort to work out your mind at least once a day.

Getting checked out if you think you're struggling with Alzheimer's

It's true that there is no cure for Alzheimer's, but there are treatments. It is important to know when you have Alzheimer's, and the sooner you can recognize the symptoms the better, because you can then work to slow the progression of the symptoms.

This goes for if you've been noticing symptoms in a loved one as well! Don't be afraid to gently broach the subject of a potential physical examination if you think you know someone whose struggling. You can be there for your friend too, you can even recommend this guide to them if they aren't sure how to handle things.

What to expect when getting checked for Alzheimer's

If you or someone you know has come in suspecting they are suffering from Alzheimer's, your doctor will do several things. They will take blood work, they may perform a physical, and they will likely administer mental tests.

These tests enable your loved ones and your medical practitioners to know where you're at, and get an idea of how best to treat you.

One such mental test they may ask you to take is the Clock Drawing Test. The clock drawing test, as the name suggests, involves asking a person to draw a clock, often one that shows a specific time.

The scorer is looking for five things to examine a person's mental state: the shape of the clock (a circle), the numbers on the clock, the order of the numbers on the clock, the hands on the clock, and whether the correct time was reflected or not.

This gives a total scoring out of five, and gives the scorer some indication of the mental state of the person who was asked to draw. Drawing has been shown to give a window of insight into a person's mental capacities, and in this case their memory (as they were asked to draw a specific time).

Conclusions

All of these tips come together to make you healthier, happier, and indeed to prevent Alzheimer's. By working to stay sharp, you will stay sharp for longer periods. This logic applies whether you're perfectly healthy or already know you have AD. Work to implement them a few at a time to ensure that you're sticking with the good habits you're trying to set, and consider the plan below if you're struggling to begin.

Making a Plan to Prevent Alzheimer's

By this point you should know what Alzheimer's is, several theories about what causes it, ways people can treat it, and ways people can prevent it.

What's next? Planning how you and your loved ones will prevent Alzheimer's of course, or delay its progression!!

I will provide a 30 day plan to get you started, but the changes you're making should be long lasting. These should be the first 30 practice days for the rest of your life, as they aim only to keep you healthy and happy while preventing Alzheimer's.

Refer back to the chapter above (our summary checklist) whenever you're making a plan of your own, and don't be afraid to look again the 30 day plan to refresh your memory of what should be changing week to week.

If You Already Have Alzheimer's, or Think You Do

Things work a little differently if you've already started to show the symptoms of Alzheimer's. If you or your loved one is already struggling with the disease, make sure that a) they get diagnosed and b) they still follow the tips from this guide!

This guide focused on prevention of Alzheimer's, that's true. However, a lot of the methods that were recommended are also effective at slowing the progression of the disease. Indeed, an antioxidant rich diet with a healthy, active lifestyle will slow your brain damage easily – and give you the precious time with loved ones that you deserve to enjoy while you can.

A study published in 2006 by the Weizmann Institute indicated that rats who were physically and mentally active in their daily life actually produced cells that were able to repair some brain damage within the hippocampus (primarily related to memory), removing some of the plaque build up and reducing the presence of toxins within their minds. This has good implications for people suffering from Alzheimer's.

The body may not be able to reverse all brain damage, but it can prevent more from happening, and slow down the ability of the disease to progress. Science is constantly looking for ways to make the path easier for those suffering from dementia and Alzheimer's, so take hope.

The same studies that have been published indicating Alzheimer's can be prevented also indicate that it can be slowed. By following the tips that have been outlined in this guide, you will be doing yourself a favour – and even improving your quality of life while you do it.

A 30 Day Plan to Preventing Alzheimer's

I recognize that there was a lot of information given to you in this guide. While I'm happy about that, I also don't want to see you so overloaded that you wind up making no changes at all to your lifestyle.

This chapter outlines a 30 day plan that implements the changes we've talked about, week by week. You can begin the rest of your life this month! Enjoy the plan, and feel free to review it if you ever start getting off track.

Week 1 – The Beginning
In this first week, I want you to head to the doctors for a physical. This physical will provide you with information about your cholesterol, your nutritional deficiencies, and gives you room to ask about a workout routine.

There's a lot of preparation that goes into changing your life, so next hit up the health food store to pick up any multivitamins or supplement needs, and out to the grocery store to make sure you're stocked with healthy food.

Remember: You could be looking for multivitamins that contain acetyl-L-carnitine (if not already in something), 400mcg of folic acid, ginkgo biloba supplements with 24% or more of flavone glycosides, hyperzine, or omega 3 fatty acid supplements with at least 1,000 mg of DHA.

Keep in mind that with all of this preparation to do good for yourself, you can still see little progress if you keep up bad habits – like smoking. If you smoke, quit. It's time. Get a patch, seek therapeutic help, and tell your friends you're done with cigarettes. Your body will thank you for it if this is the only thing you do.

Week 2 – Here We Go

If the focus of the first week was getting a baseline, the focus of the second week is implementing changes. At this point your kitchen should be stocked with whole grains, antioxidants, and fruits and veggies. If it's not, head back out to the grocery store.

Also, have your water checked. If your tap water is high in aluminum, replace it with bottled. Staying hydrated is key to your health, and avoiding aluminum is key to this plan. The body does not do well dehydrated, and it does not do well when chalk full of aluminum.

Try making a meal plan if you're struggling with your diet, as planning ahead will help you to ensure you're getting everything you need – and make your shopping trip easier to boot.

Week 3

This is where we begin to focus on the body, your physique. Make sure you've begun exercising. Recall that you don't need a gym membership or bill from the department store to work out, you can do it yourself, with simple routines.

You should be working out between 3-5 times a week in 20-30 minute sessions of heart pumping fun. Try aerobics, bicycling, sit-ups, or other basic things to see changes take effect.

If you are currently out of shape, don't let this stop you. It's not too late. Just make sure you've cleared your routine with a health professional (so you don't push too hard to quickly) and start implementing this routine.

Week 4

This is the final week, everything should be in place and pulled together. You're eating better, you're more active, and you're tracking your progress. By now you should be well on your way to the kind of lifestyle that prevents Alzheimer's.

Congratulations! And keep it up!

Beyond Week 4

You may have noticed that a lot of time in that first month is spent in planning as well as in action. This is because this plan, the tips in this guide, are meant to make lifelong meaningful changes for you. After week 4 you don't just cross your fingers and assume you're done, you continue to work on your progress.

Keep eating well. Stay active. Work out your brain! If you follow these tips, you will be keeping your mind safe and healthy as long as humanly possible.

Tracking Your Progress

As you're going through these changes, keep a little daily log of how you're doing. Include whether you exercised, how you exercised, and how long you did it for. Include whether or not you ate well, and if not, why not.

Keeping track of your progress helps you in two ways. One, it functions as an accountability tool, keeping yourself accountable so you can see when you've slipped and strategically plan about how to fix it.

The other way that it helps though is more subtle, this can be an encouraging log! As you see yourself keeping up with your diet, or exercising more often, you will be constantly reminding yourself of the good work you've already done – which keeps you motivated to keep doing it.

Conclusions

We've probably all heard the saying "you are as young as you think you are". The guidelines in this book are set in place to help you keep yourself younger, for longer. The aging process can seem daunting and scary, but rest assured that with the tips from this guide you are already doing all you can to combat age related declines.

There's no reason to fear one year more than the next when you know you've done all you can to enable yourself to enjoy it and live it well.

Visit :
www.naturesnaturalhealth.com/join/
To Sign Up for our Exclusive Health Newsletter TODAY!

www.ingramcontent.com/pod-product-compliance
Lightning Source LLC
Chambersburg PA
CBHW060640290526
45793CB00001B/334